REVERSE BACK AND SHOULDER PAIN

Effective Home Exercises for Relieving Back and Shoulder Pain

Reverse Your Pain Series
Book 3

Morgan Sutherland, L.M.T.

Reverse Back and Shoulder Pain

Effective Home Exercises for Relieving
Back and Shoulder Pain

Reverse Your Pain Series Book 3

Copyright © 2019 Morgan Sutherland, L.M.T.

All rights reserved.

ISBN: 979-8-9864227-4-9

Illustrations: Copyright Morgan Sutherland

Cover image: 123RF

CONTENTS

MEDICAL DISCLAIMER

The information provided in this book is not intended to be a substitute for professional medical advice, diagnosis, or treatment. Never disregard or delay seeking professional medical advice because of something you read in this book. Never rely on information in this book in place of seeking professional medical advice.

Morgan Sutherland is not responsible or liable for any advice, course of treatment, diagnosis, other information, services, and/or products that you obtain in this book. You are encouraged to consult with your doctor or healthcare provider with regard to the information contained in this book. After reading this book, you are encouraged to review the information carefully with your professional healthcare provider.

PERSONAL DISCLAIMER

I am not a doctor. The information I provide is based on my personal experiences and research as a licensed massage therapist. Any recommendations I make about posture, exercise, stretching, and massage should be discussed with your professional healthcare provider to prevent any risk to your health.

INTRODUCTION

Recently, I was at a popular burrito joint waiting for my order, so I naturally started observing the other customers' gait and posture.

I'll admit that it's hard to maintain perfect sitting posture while devouring a classic Mexican burrito.

However, I couldn't help but notice a handful of people who succumbed to gravity and slumped over their sumptuous burritos with Quasimodo-like hunchback posture.

Poor posture can lead to knots galore, especially in the back.

Eight out of every ten people experience back pain at some time in their lives.

Many of my back pain clients come into my office complaining of knots in their upper back, especially between their shoulder blades.

Stubborn knots or neck cricks, as some people call them, can make looking over your shoulder annoyingly tricky and painful.

Why is it when you sleep all twisted up like a pretzel, you awake wishing you had a four-year-old's Gumby flexible neck?

When your neck is bent to one side for an extended time, the muscles and ligaments stretch and can keep pulling to the point of tearing.

It can be a mild or a severe tear, and the resulting pain and limited movement can last for a day or two or for several weeks.

Not fun!

The body's natural reaction to any contracted area with poor circulation is to lay down connective tissue (also known as collagen fibers, the building blocks of scar tissue).

Despite the healing nature of this process, it inevitably "glues" muscles and their connective tissue coverings into a shortened state, limiting the range of motion of joints and body parts.

However, when the knot is more serious, you'll feel that your neck is sore, and there's muscle pain in your shoulder blade on the same side.

Can Massage Help Get Rid of Knots in Your Back?

Yes! Massage is a conversation with your nervous system. Applying the right amount of pressure on a trigger point (a sensitive spot in the muscle area) for 10 seconds to a minute can soften the muscle tension and coax the nervous system to relax.

You can try self-massaging your knots with a tennis ball or a trigger point tool, or you can schedule a professional massage.

Massage is just part of the puzzle in reversing back and shoulder pain.

The other main tool to master is building a healthy habit of performing regular corrective exercises that combat the symptoms of bad posture, so you don't end up looking like the hunched-over supervillain Gru from Despicable Me.

UPPER CROSSED SYNDROME AND HOW TO FIX IT

The phenomenon of text neck, also referred to as upper crossed syndrome, has become a frequent ailment and seems like it's unavoidable. Nearly everybody slumps their head to look at their smartphone. The next time you do, consider these facts . . .

The weight of the average head is equal to that of a bowling ball. As a person lets gravity take over, his or her cervical spine absorbs the brunt of that added weight.

At a 15-degree angle, this weight equates to about 27 pounds; at 30 degrees it's 40 pounds; and when it reaches 60 degrees that's **60 pounds of pressure on your neck**.

Sustained forward head posture overstretches the neck muscles, leaving them sore and inflamed. Not only can text neck cause muscle strains, pinched nerves, and herniated disks, but over time it can even erase the neck's natural curve.

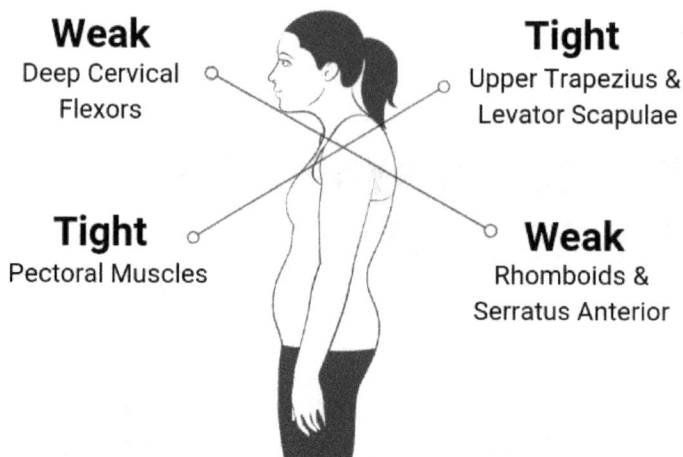

Weak
Deep Cervical
Flexors

Tight
Upper Trapezius &
Levator Scapulae

Tight
Pectoral Muscles

Weak
Rhomboids &
Serratus Anterior

Upper crossed syndrome is a pattern of muscular imbalances and postural distortions in the head, neck, and upper shoulders.

These imbalances can occur when muscles are continuously tightened and shortened or overstretched and weakened.

This condition is given its name because an X (in other words, crossed) can be drawn across the upper body.

Specifically, the muscles at the back of the neck and shoulders (upper trapezius and levator scapulae) become incredibly tight. The muscles in the front of the neck and chest (sternocleidomastoid and the pectoralis major and minor muscles) also become tight.

As a result of these overly tight muscles, the surrounding counter muscles become overstretched and weakened.

This reciprocal muscle weakness occurs in the deep cervical flexors (anterior neck muscles), lower trapezius, and serratus anterior.

Common Characteristics of Upper Crossed Syndrome

- Forward head posture
- Increased cervical lordosis (curvature in the spine of the neck vertebrae)
- Increased thoracic kyphosis (rounded upper back and shoulders)
- Elevated, protracted, or rounded shoulders

Common Symptoms of Upper Crossed Syndrome

- Headache
- Neck pain and stiffness
- Greater susceptibility to neck strains in the back of the neck and weakness in the front
- Chest pain and tightness
- Upper back pain (especially knots in the shoulder blades)
- Restricted range of motion in the neck or shoulders
- Pain, numbness, and tingling down the upper arms into the fingers
- Lower back pain

In this book, you will learn step-by-step corrective exercises to fix upper crossed syndrome and lower back pain, so you can live a healthier and more harmonious life.

https://www.ncbi.nlm.nih.gov/pubmed/31040591

https://www.healthline.com/health/upper-crossed-syndrome

THREE POSTURAL STRESSES THAT MESS UP YOUR SHOULDERS

Nurturing poor postural habits, such as working or hanging out in a slouched position, can make the shoulders rounded and the head more forward.

This postural neglect can ultimately make it more challenging to move the shoulders back into proper alignment.

Too much wear and tear on your shoulder region will inevitably weaken the shoulder muscles, known as the rotator cuff, and make them less flexible and more prone to injury.

The rotator cuff muscles can become overstretched, overloaded, and injured when you vigorously pull something, like weeds, or lift and haul a heavy suitcase.

A direct fall on the shoulder, elbow, or hand can undoubtedly cause serious harm.

1. Raised Arm Postures

Performing repetitive or prolonged tasks with raised arm positions (above shoulder height) can gradually overstretch, overload, or compress the shoulder structure.

Solution A: Try to adopt positions where your arms or elbows are close to your body—either by your side or in front of you.

Solution B: Perform activities for a shorter amount of time. Every 10 minutes or so, take a 30-second break.

This will let the shoulder muscle recover and help build a healthy habit of pacing your activities.

Solution C: Take a stretch break. Stand upright, clasp your hands behind your back and try to pull your shoulder blades together.

Hold for 3 seconds.

Repeat five times.

2. Sitting in a Slouched Position for a Prolonged Period

During sitting, the position of your low back has a strong influence on your neck and shoulder posture.

If the low back is allowed to slouch, your neck and shoulders will be following suit.

The head slowly juts forward, the shoulders become rounded, and the rotator cuff muscles become overstretched and fatigued (weakening them).

Solution: Put a lumbar roll at the small of your back about waist level to support your low back. This will create a natural hollow (lordosis) that is present when you're standing.

3. Lying Down and Sleeping

Waking in the morning with a stiff and painful shoulder that wasn't bothering you the night before could most likely be caused by poor sleep postures.

Lying in a position that puts unwanted stress on the shoulder, like lying on it or lying in a raised-arm posture, can gradually overstretch and strain the rotator cuff muscles.

If you already have a painful shoulder, then poor sleeping postures can exasperate the pain.

Solution A: Don't sleep on the painful shoulder for any length of time. Try a larger or more supportive pillow, while maintaining normal alignment of the neck.

Solution B: Sleep on your back, with a pillow underneath your painful shoulder, or sleep on the nonpainful side

UPPER CROSSED SYNDROME EXERCISE ROUTINE

A 2017 study published in the *Journal of Physical Therapy Science* aimed to determine the effect of forward head posture-improving exercises on rounded shoulder posture.

The research featured the benefits of (1) the McKenzie Method (an approach to assessment and treatment) and the use of repeat movements, (2) implementing a stretching regimen, and (3) utilizing the Kendall strengthening physical therapy exercises.

These three proven techniques were compared side by side to determine which had the most significant positive impact on the symptoms associated with posture-related injuries.

The results revealed that all three techniques had a strikingly similar effect on decreasing the symptoms associated with these injuries, specifically those related to rounded shoulders and forward head postures.

The following eleven neck and shoulder exercises blend both McKenzie's neck-stretching protocol with Kendall's strengthening exercises.

https://www.ncbi.nlm.nih.gov/pmc/articles/PMC5684019/

1. Chin Tuck

The head retraction exercise (commonly referred to as chin tuck) can help reverse forward head posture by strengthening the neck muscles. This exercise can be done sitting or standing.

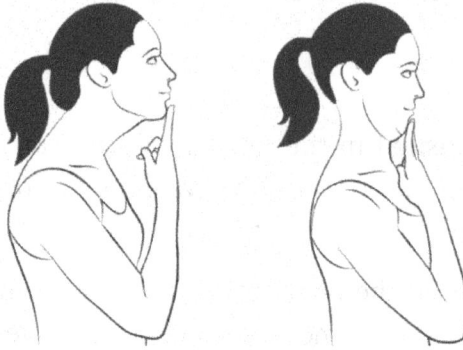

Start with your shoulders rolled back and down. While looking straight ahead, place two fingers on your chin, slightly tuck your chin, and move your head back.

Hold for 3 to 5 seconds and then release.

Repeat ten times.

2. Neck Extension (Part 1)

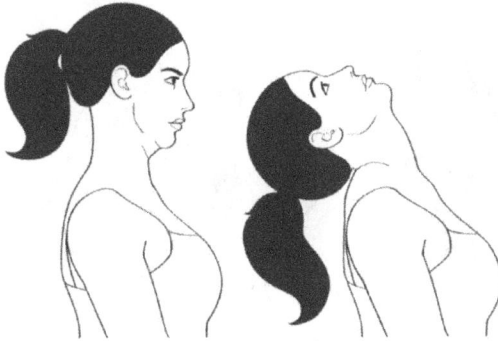

While holding your head in the chin tuck position, raise your chin and tilt your head backward, looking upward.

Make sure to not let your neck move forward during this exercise.

Neck Extension (Part 2)

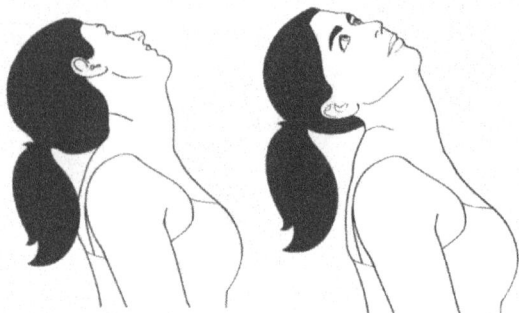

While your head is tilted back, rotate your head side to side. Strive to steadily move your head and neck farther back as you turn.

Hold the stretch for a few seconds.

Repeat ten times.

Repeat in the opposite direction.

3. Neck Lateral Flexion (Part 1)

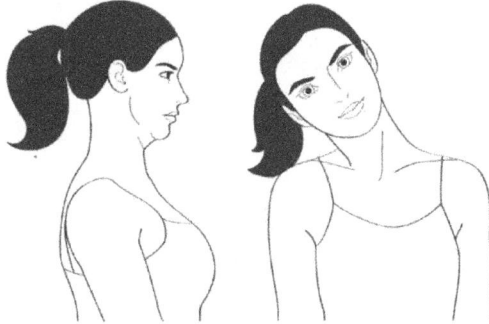

Look straight ahead and begin with the chin tuck exercise.

Then move your right ear toward your right shoulder.

Neck Lateral Flexion (Part 2)

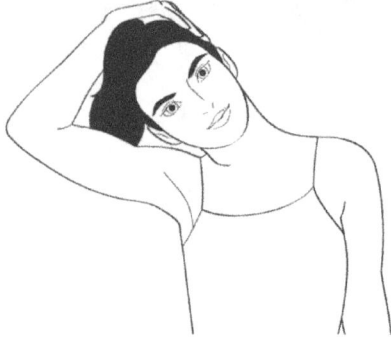

To make this stretch more effective, drape the hand of your most painful side over your head, above your ear, and pull your head even farther toward the painful side.

Hold the stretch for a few seconds.

Repeat ten times.

Repeat on the opposite side.

4. Neck Rotation (Part 1)

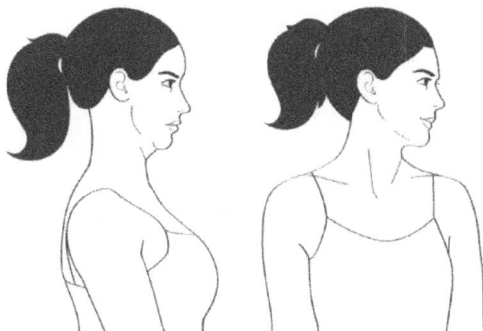

Start by looking straight ahead and performing the chin tuck exercise.

Then look over your left shoulder as far as you can.

If one side feels more painful, rotate toward that side.

Hold for a few seconds, and then move your head back to the midline. If neck pain doesn't decrease after a few rotations, then rotate toward the least painful side.

Repeat ten times.

Then rotate toward the other side.

Neck Rotation (Part 2)

To take your neck rotation up a notch, use both your hands to gently push your head farther into the rotation.

Hold the stretch for a few seconds.

Return to the start position.

Repeat ten times.

Then switch sides.

5. Neck Flexion

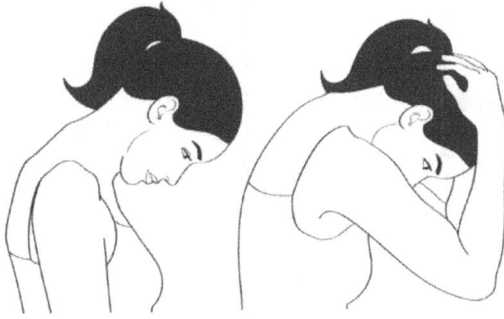

Start by placing the head and neck in a midline position. Bend the head forward until the chin touches the chest.

When it is difficult to reach the chest, flex the neck as far as it can go without pain.

Hold for a few seconds.

Then move the head back to the start position.

Repeat this stretch ten times.

6. Wall Angels

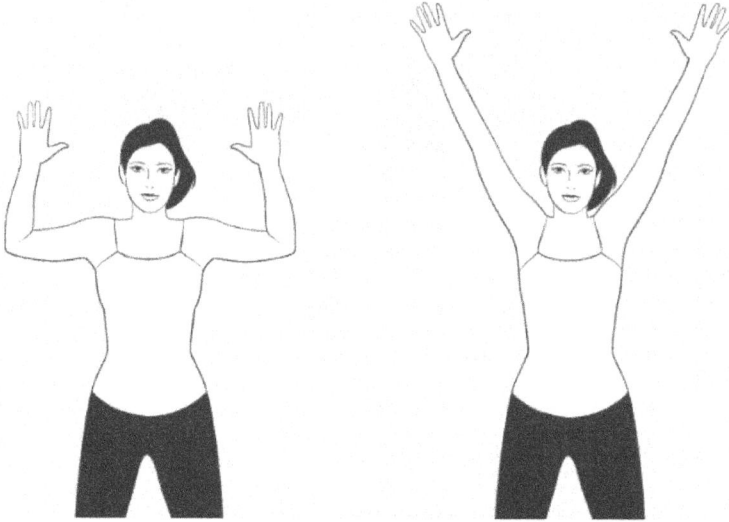

Keep your feet about 4 inches away from the wall and maintain a slight bend in your knees. Your glutes (muscles in your buttocks), spine, and head should all be against the wall as you move the shoulder blades together and squeeze, forming the letter "W" with your arms. Hold for 3 seconds.

Now, raise your arms to form the letter "Y." Make sure not to shrug your shoulders to your ears. Repeat ten times, starting at "W," holding for 3 seconds, and then raising your arms into a "Y." Do two to three sets.

7. Doorway Stretch (Part 1): Pectoralis Stretch

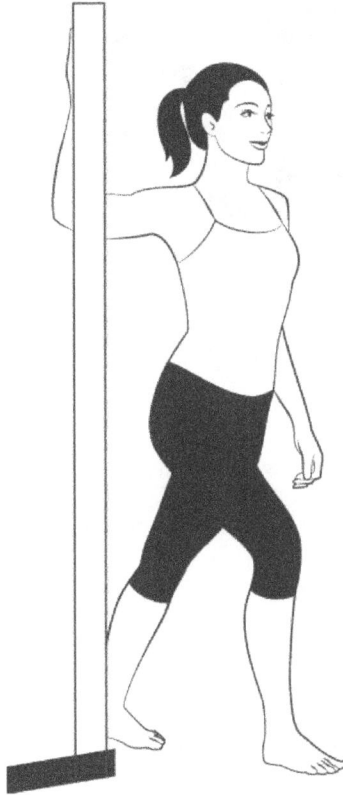

This exercise helps to loosen tight chest muscles.

First, reach your arm outward 90 degrees. Then, place your hand on the doorjamb and lean forward.

Slowly, lean into your raised arm and push against the doorjamb for 7 to 10 seconds.

Relax and then stretch your bent arm back and stretch your chest for 7 to 10 seconds.

Repeat this stretch two to three times.

Doorway Stretch (Part 2): Subscapularis Stretch

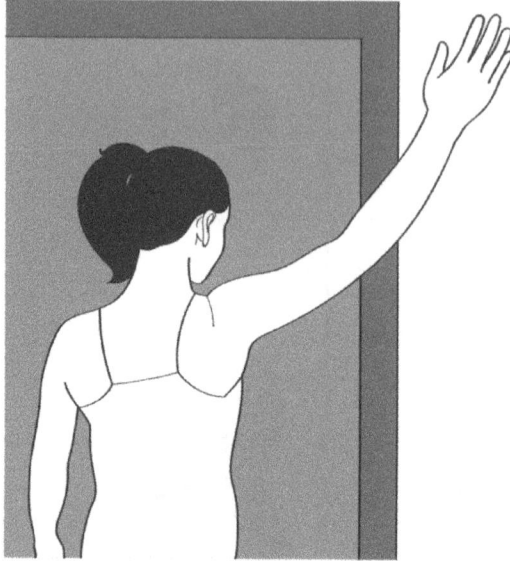

Raise your arm higher along the doorjamb so that it's at a 45-degree angle.

Slowly, lean into your raised arm and push against the doorjamb for 7 to 10 seconds.

Relax and then stretch your bent arm back. Stretch your chest for 7 to 10 seconds.

Repeat this stretch two to three times.

https://www.youtube.com/watch?v=bMkp_0BtLQg

8. Shoulder Extension

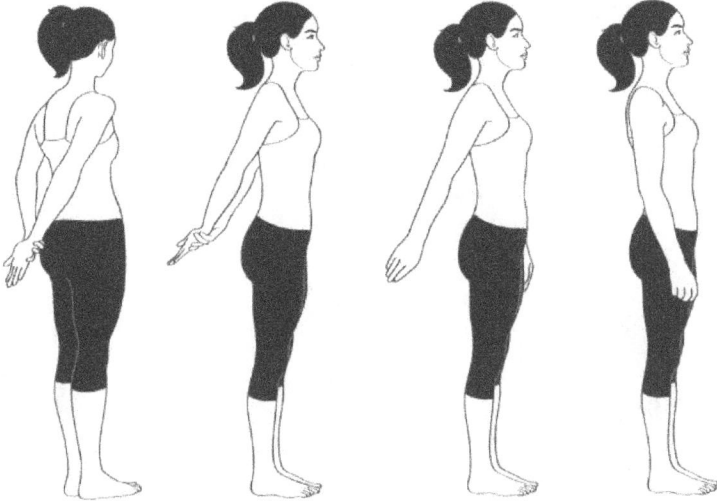

Stand upright with your head in a neutral position.

With your nonpainful arm, grasp the wrist of your painful arm. Pull it away from your back until you feel a good stretch in your sore shoulder.

Hold the stretch for a few seconds.

Then return to the starting position.

Repeat ten times, each time trying to move your shoulder back farther.

9. Bent over L

The bent over L exercise works your shoulders and upper back muscles.

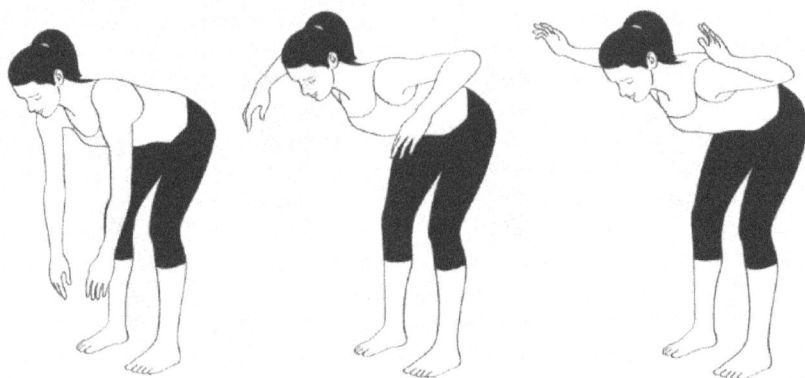

Begin by bending over at the waist with your hips, back, and knees slightly bent.

While maintaining a flat back and raised chest, glide your shoulder blades back and down, and then lift your elbows toward the ceiling, as you bend them to 90 degrees.

When your elbows reach shoulder height, rotate your forearms upward, until the backs of your hands are facing the ceiling.

Reverse this pattern back to the starting position and repeat for 10 repetitions. Do three sets.

10. Bent over Thoracic Rotation

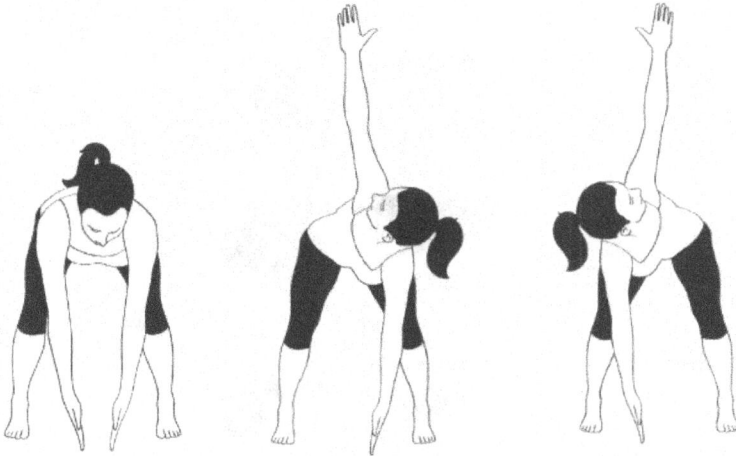

Start in a standing position. Bend over with a good neutral spine position. Then follow your hand with your eyes as you rotate up toward the ceiling.

Make sure to move entirely through your upper back, keeping your hips and belly button level to the ground the entire time.

Alternate rotating up to the left and right. Do three sets of 10 rotations.

https://www.youtube.com/watch?v=NF9OwEYu1JE

11. Prone YTW Exercise

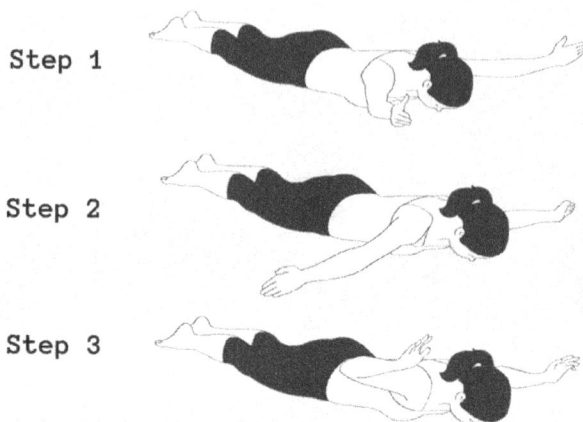

Step 1

Step 2

Step 3

Step 1: The Y

Lie on your stomach (preferably on a mat), gently exhale, and slowly lift your arms off the floor, moving your arms into a Y formation, with palms facing inward.

Keep your head aligned with your upper spine. Focus on lifting from the shoulders and not the low back.

Hold this position for 1 to 2 seconds.

Then relax and return to your starting position.

Repeat ten times.

Step 2: The T

From the same starting position, gently exhale, and slowly lift your arms off the floor, moving your arms into the T formation, as illustrated, with palms facing forward.

Hold this position for 1 to 2 seconds, then relax and return to your starting position.

Repeat ten times.

Step 3: The W

Gently exhale, and slowly lift your arms off the floor. Bend your elbows and pull them toward your waist, forming the letter W with your palms facing inward.

Hold this position for 1 to 2 seconds.

Then relax and return to your starting position.

Repeat ten times.

https://www.youtube.com/watch?v=3MxHX9j15BU

SEVEN RESISTANCE BAND EXERCISES FOR CORRECTING ROUNDED SHOULDERS

When I hear the words "bad posture," there are two things that immediately come to mind. First is **forward head posture**, and second is **rounded shoulders**.

As you lean closer to your computer monitor and your shoulders begin to slouch, you subconsciously adjust your head position and fix your gaze to look straight.

This leads to a muscular imbalance and excessive shortening of the posterior head and neck muscles, forcing the upper neck bones to protrude forward, resulting in rounded shoulders and rounded back.

To reverse the skeletal defects of this hunched look and improve your upper body posture, you must first focus on **two essential things.**

1. Stretching your pectoral muscles (chest muscles).

2. Strengthening your posterior scapular stabilizers (upper back and shoulder muscles; your trapezius, rhomboids, and levator scapulae).

Doorway Pectoralis Stretch

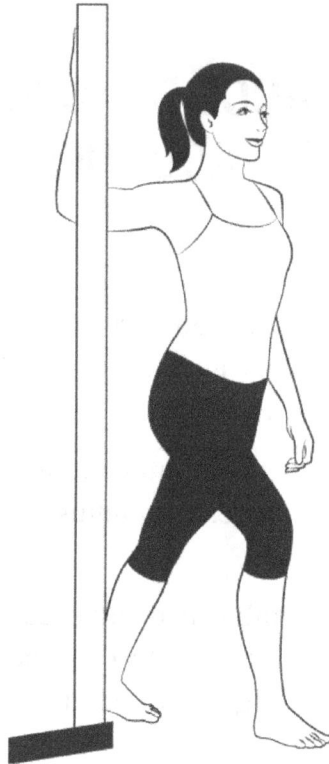

This exercise helps to loosen tight chest muscles.

First, reach your arm outward 90 degrees. Then, place your hand on the doorjamb and lean forward.

Slowly, lean into your raised arm and push against the doorjamb for 7 to 10 seconds.

Relax and then stretch your bent arm back and stretch your chest for 7 to 10 seconds.

Repeat this stretch two to three times.

Doorway Subscapularis Stretch

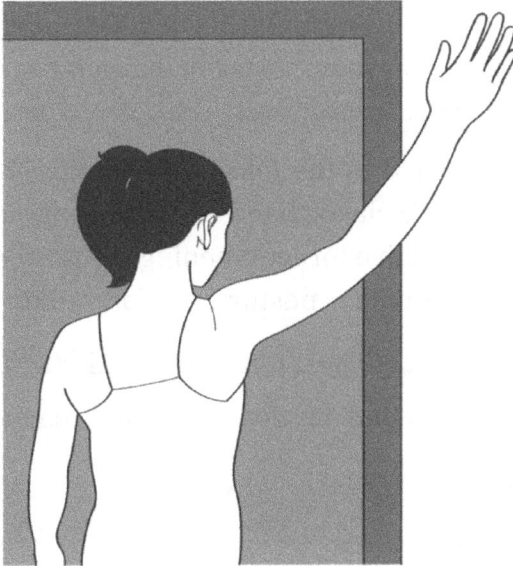

The subscapularis muscle is one of the four rotator cuff muscles, located deep in the armpit on the anterior portion of the scapulae.

Muscular adhesions and trigger points in the subscapularis can lead to pain and restricted shoulder movement.

To stretch the subscapularis muscle, raise your arm to 45 degrees on the doorjamb and lean forward.

Slowly, lean into your raised arm and push against the doorjamb for 7 to 10 seconds.

Relax and then stretch your bent arm back and stretch your chest for 7 to 10 seconds.

Repeat this stretch two to three times.

https://www.huffpost.com/entry/frozen-shoulder_b_1733786

Correct Rounded Shoulders with These Seven Resistance Band Exercises

In order to strengthen your posterior scapular stabilizers, you'll need resistance bands.

A 2016 study published in the *Journal of Physical Therapy Science* found that a resistance elastic band exercise program consisting of seven moves was effective for lengthening the pectoralis major and correcting rounded shoulder posture and forward head posture.

https://www.ncbi.nlm.nih.gov/pmc/articles/PMC4932046/

In this section, you can find all seven resistance band exercises.

Repeat fifteen times per set.

Do three sets in total.

Move 1: Lat Pull Down

The muscles of the upper back are vital to maintain good posture and shoulder stabilization. This area is prone to dysfunction because of poor posture associated with rounded backs.

The lat pull down exercise helps to strengthen and reverse the harmful effects of this postural distortion.

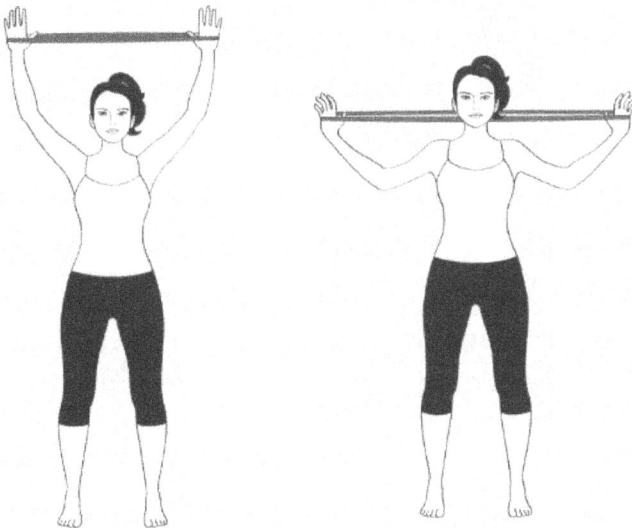

Begin by grasping a medium resistance band loop around each hand

Raise it above your head.

Next, pull down the band and push out at the same time.

Hold for 2 seconds and slowly return.

Repeat eight to twelve times.

Do three sets.

http://www.performancehealthacademy.com/thera-band-loop-lat-pull-down.html

35

Move 2: Resisted External Rotation

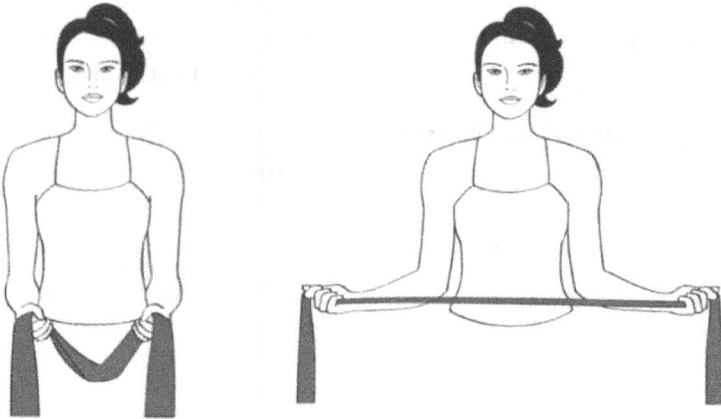

With your arms by your sides and the elbows bent at a 90-degree angle, hold the resistance band between your hands with your palms facing up.

Move your hands apart to rotate your shoulders while squeezing the shoulder blades together down and back.

Repeat eight to twelve times.

Do three sets.

https://www.youtube.com/watch?v=4tpl-huz060

Move 3: Shoulder Horizontal Abduction

Extend your arms in front of your body at a 90-degree angle, shoulder-width apart.

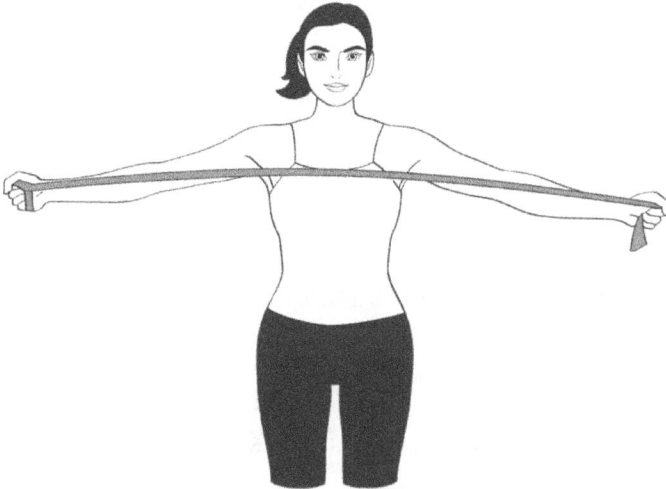

Keep your palms face down as you hold the resistance band.

Now, stretch the resistance band horizontally while making sure to keep your elbows straight.

Repeat eight to twelve times.

Do three sets.

Move 4: TheraBand Row (Standing)

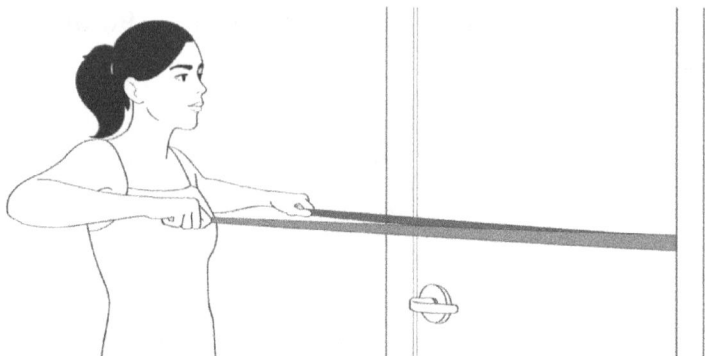

Begin standing upright, holding both ends of a resistance band (also known as a TheraBand) that is anchored in front of you at chest height, with your palms facing inward.

Pull your arms back, then return to the starting position.

Repeat eight to twelve times.

Do three sets.

Tip: Make sure to keep your core engaged and focus on squeezing your shoulder blades together as you pull on the band.

Move 5: Shoulder Abduction

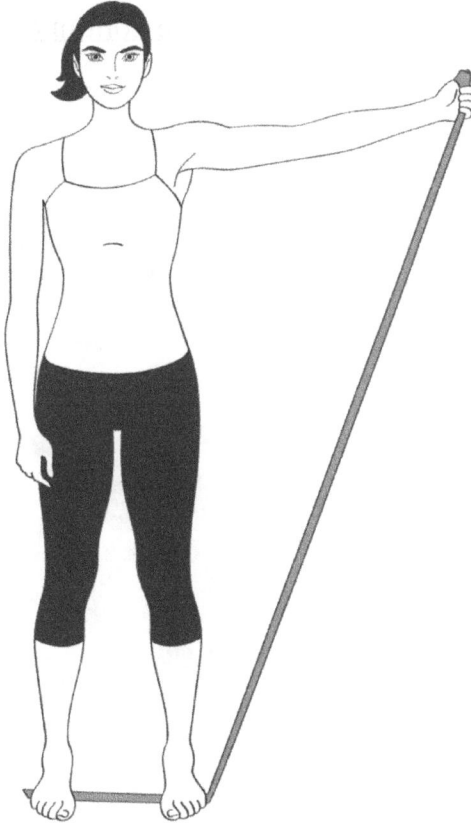

Step on the resistance band with the foot on the same side being exercised.

Now, hold the resistance band with one hand, and keep the hand low in a neutral position.

Then, abduct the shoulder by moving it out to the side with the elbow slightly bent and thumb facing up.

Take the arm, in a controlled fashion, to the end range or just before pain is felt.

Repeat eight to twelve times.

Do three sets.

https://www.youtube.com/watch?time_continue=24&v=BW0Olzz
otBI

Move 6: Shoulder Flexion

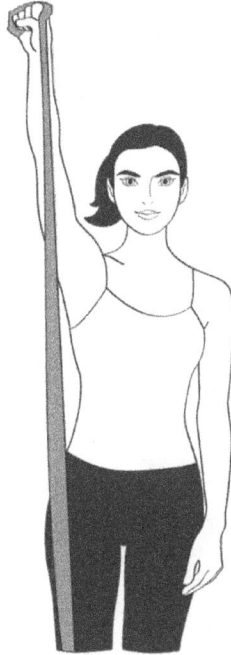

Step on the resistance band with the foot on the same side being exercised.

Now, held the resistance band with one hand, and keep the hand low in a neutral position.

Then, bend the arm forward with the elbow straightened.

Take it to the end range or just before pain is felt.

Hold and slowly return.

Repeat eight to twelve times

Do three sets.

Move 7: Shoulder Extension

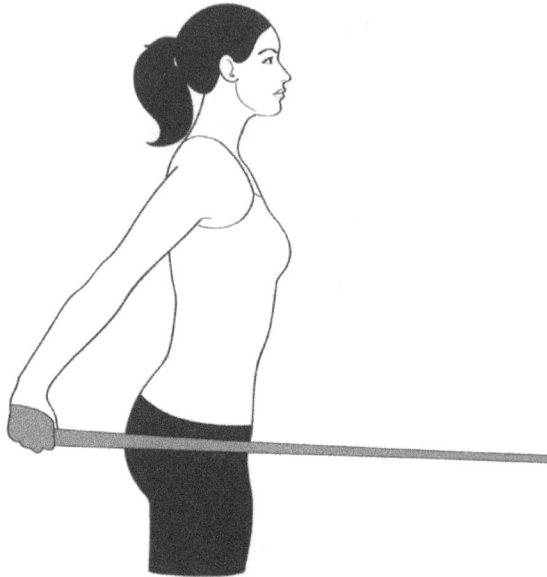

If you have someone to help, have that person hold one end of the resistance band, and you hold the other end of the resistance band. If you're alone, wrap the resistance band around a doorknob or something that won't move.

Hold the resistance band low in its neutral position.

Then, extend the arm backward, with the elbow straightened as much as possible.

Hold and slowly return.

Repeat eight to twelve times.

Do three sets.

Thoughts

You should be noticing improved posture with less slouching and rounding of the shoulders.

Practice these resistance band exercises three to four times per week, and soon people will be complimenting you on your ideal posture.

The biggest favor you can give them is to share these powerful tips about how to get rid of rounded shoulders.

HOW TO MELT STUBBORN KNOTS BETWEEN THE SHOULDER BLADES

Plugging away at your computer all day, with forward head posture, rounded shoulders, and slouched low back, is a perfect recipe for developing deep knots between your shoulder blades.

No worries! I have eight simple moves that will solve your stiff neck problems and restore your limited range of motion.

These eight super effective ways will help get rid of those stubborn knots and leave you feeling loose and pain free.

More often than not, the pain between your shoulder blades is cervicogenic, meaning that it's coming from your neck. So, the first thing you should try for relief is neck extension.

1. Neck Extension

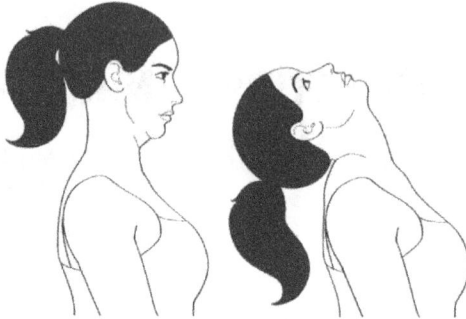

While holding your head in the chin tuck position, raise your chin and tilt your head backward, looking upward. Make sure to not let your neck move forward during this exercise.

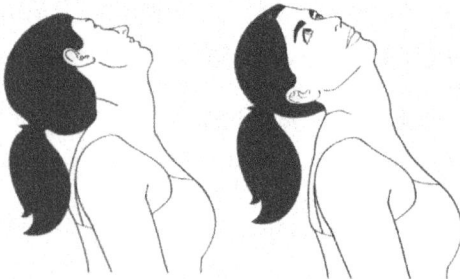

While your head is tilted back, rotate your head side to side. Strive to steadily move your head and neck farther back as you turn.

2. Towel Stretch

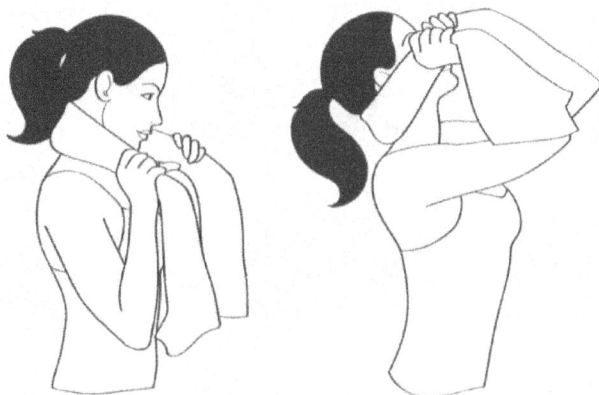

Grab a rolled-up towel or a T-shirt. Place it behind your neck just above the boniest point (called the occiput). Make sure your ears are in line with your shoulders.

Now create tension by pulling the towel forward and away from you.

Slowly raise your head, for about two breaths, keeping that tension while slowly moving the towel up.

Next, extend the neck a bit farther while maintaining the towel tension for about five breaths. Then return to a neutral neck position for two breaths.

http://www.functionalsportstherapy.com/resetting-text-neck/

3. Lacrosse Ball Arm Circles

Stretching is not enough when it comes to releasing a knotted muscle.

A cost-effective alternative to a professional deep-tissue massage is the do-it-yourself method with a tennis ball, a lacrosse ball, or a foam roller.

Lie on the floor and place the lacrosse ball right behind your shoulder blade where the tension resides.

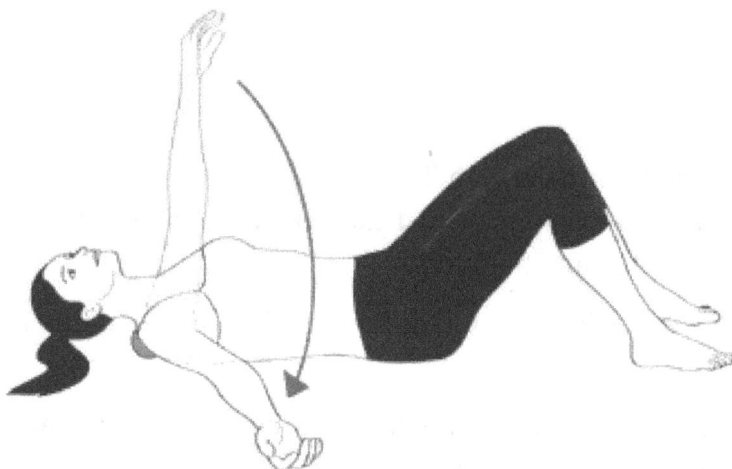

Move your arm into the air and then bring it down toward the floor as you swoop the arm around. Feel the lacrosse ball knead and gradually melt that stubborn knot between your shoulder blades.

Do ten slow arm circles.

https://www.youtube.com/watch?v=yY-7CXAHxfY

4. Foam Roll: Spinal Release

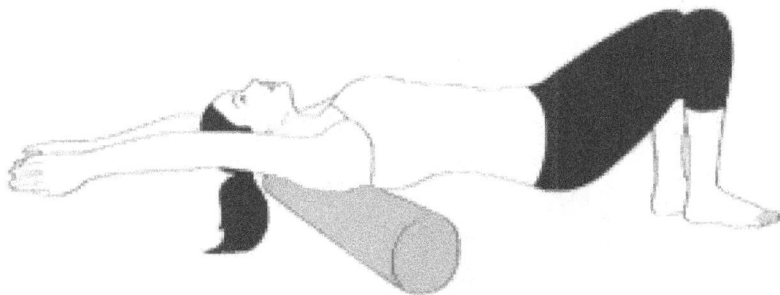

With this foam roller stretch, you won't be rolling at all; you'll be using your arms for the movement.

Lie on the floor with your shoulders over a foam roller. Bend your knees with your feet flat on the floor.

Place your arms down at your sides.

Keeping them completely straight, lift them over your head until they are touching the floor behind you (like you're raising your arms in excitement).

You can also raise them sideways, mimicking a snow-angel type of movement.

5. Foam Roll: Punch the Sky

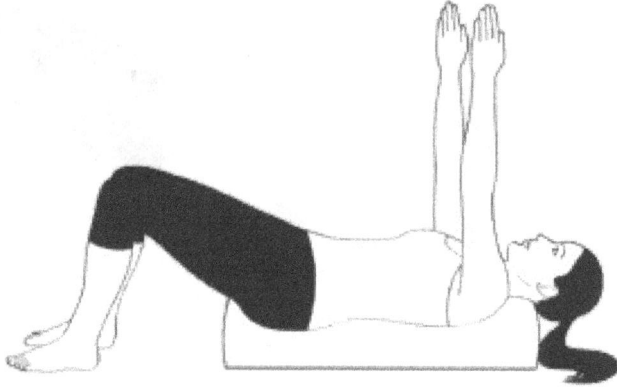

Lie vertically on the foam roller, with your arms extended out toward the ceiling, aligned with your shoulders.

Slowly reach your right arm toward the ceiling as far as you can, leaving the left arm extended and relaxed.

Now, alternate arms and reach your left arm toward the ceiling as far as you can, leaving the right arm extended and relaxed.

Once you've completed alternating from one arm to the next, "punch" both arms forward together ten times, reaching as far as you can toward the ceiling.

6. Thread the Needle

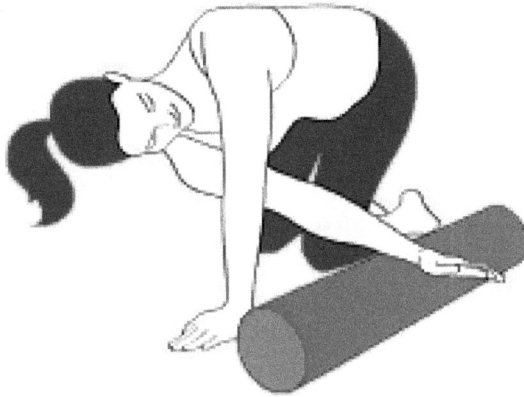

If the foam roller is along your left side (see the above illustration), reach your right arm under your body and place it palm up on the foam roller.

Push your right arm forward so that your body begins to twist, and the foam roller begins to roll toward your elbow. Follow your arm with your head.

Roll back to the center position.

Repeat five times.

Turn your head away from your arm.

Repeat five times.

Flip your hand over, palm down.

Repeat five times with your head toward your arm.

51

Repeat five times with your head away from your arm.

Switch the foam roller to the opposite side.

Repeat.

Note: Only go as far as you're comfortable while doing this stretch.

7. Cat and Cow Pose

Starting on your hands and knees, an all-fours position, move into the Cat Pose by slowly pressing your spine up, arching your back.

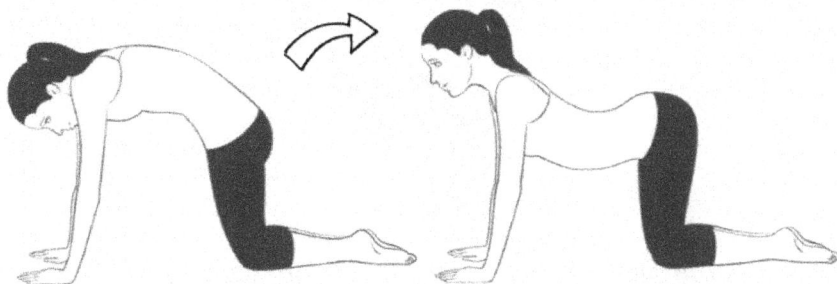

Hold the pose for a few seconds, and then move to the Cow Pose by scooping your spine in, pressing your shoulder blades back and lifting your head. Moving back and forth from Cat Pose to Cow Pose helps move your spine to a neutral position, relaxing the muscles and easing tension.

Repeat the sequence ten times, flowing smoothly from cat to cow, and cow back to cat.

8. Spinal Twist

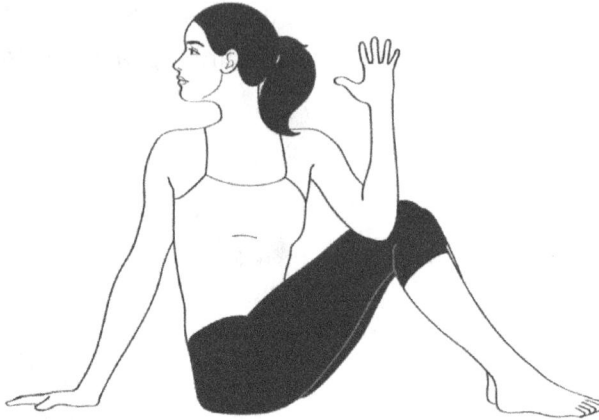

Twisting from your thoracic spine (middle spine), where your shoulder blades are, will help to stretch the stiffness in a rounded upper back.

Sit on the floor, with your knees up and feet flat.

Twist your body to the right. Place your right arm behind you with your palm down.

Take a deep breath and, as you exhale, place your left elbow on the outside of your right knee.

Push into your knee, twisting into the stretch.

https://www.doyouyoga.com/6-yoga-poses-to-correct-rounded-shoulders-and-relieve-pain-53703/

THE SECRET TO THAWING OUT A FROZEN SHOULDER

In this section, you're going to learn the secret to thawing out a frozen shoulder. I'll be discussing the causes, common signs, and surgery-free ways to treat this debilitating pain condition.

If you simply can't raise your arm past your ears without excruciating pain, then there's a good chance you might have a frozen shoulder.

Frozen shoulder, also known as adhesive capsulitis, is when the shoulder is painful and loses its full range of motion due to inflammation.

What Causes a Frozen Shoulder?

The shoulder joint rests in a capsule, like a ball and socket.

Ligaments secure the shoulder bones to each other.

When the joint becomes inflamed, as from an injury, lack of exercise, or previous surgery, the shoulder bones become unable to move freely in the joint.

WHAT ARE THE COMMON SIGNS OF A FROZEN SHOULDER?

Pain, lack of movement, and stiffness when moving your arm are some clear signs of a frozen shoulder.

Over time, sleeping is severely affected, and it becomes nearly impossible to perform activities, such as reaching over your head or behind you.

Note: Don't try to self-diagnose your shoulder pain.

It's best to go to your primary healthcare provider and get a full assessment about a stiff, painful shoulder. This might include X-rays, an ultrasound, or an MRI to rule out other problems.

HOW LONG CAN A SHOULDER STAY FROZEN?

There are three phases to a frozen shoulder. The freezing phase, the frozen phase, and the thawing out phase.

Phase 1: Freezing

On average the freezing phase, which is characterized by constant pain and limited range of motion, can last between two and nine months or up to a year.

Phase 2: Frozen

The frozen phase is when the shoulder stiffness gradually increases, and this can go on for another twelve months.

Phase 3: Thawing Out

The thawing-out phase is a sign of a road to recovery, with the shoulder functionality improving and the pain easing. This improvement can take between twelve and twenty-four months.

For approximately 80 percent of frozen shoulder patients, the pain disappears and their range of motion returns. However, some will experience permanently restricted range of motion. This loss of motion does not usually cause any long-term problems.

TWO SURGERY-FREE WAYS TO TREAT A FROZEN SHOULDER

1. Cortisone shots into the shoulder joint might offer short-term relief.

2. Physical therapy and massage therapy can be effective in improving the range of motion of a frozen shoulder problem.

That said, I had a massage client who came to me with a frozen shoulder, and it took her a little over a year to regain 90 percent mobility.

She was definitely on the road to recovery when she ended treatment.

It just takes patience.

Doing physical therapy exercises at home can help keep your shoulder mobile and strong, so you can avoid further stiffness.

SEVEN FROZEN SHOULDER EXERCISES

The following seven frozen shoulder exercises are recommended by Harvard Medical School.

Before beginning a frozen shoulder exercise routine, it's best to warm up your shoulders.

A 10 to 15-minute warm shower or bath will suffice. Or use a moist heat pad, but the latter might not be as effective.

When performing the following shoulder exercises, it's always wise to stretch to the point of tension but not pain.

1. Pendulum Stretch

Begin by relaxing your affected shoulder, leaning over slightly and letting your arm hang down. Draw small circles in the air with your hand.

Perform ten circles in a clockwise direction and then ten circles in a counterclockwise direction.

Perform this once a day. As your symptoms improve, gently increase the diameter of your swing while drawing circles in the air.

Once this pendulum exercise feels easy, increase the stretch by holding a light weight (3 to 5 pounds) in your swinging arm.

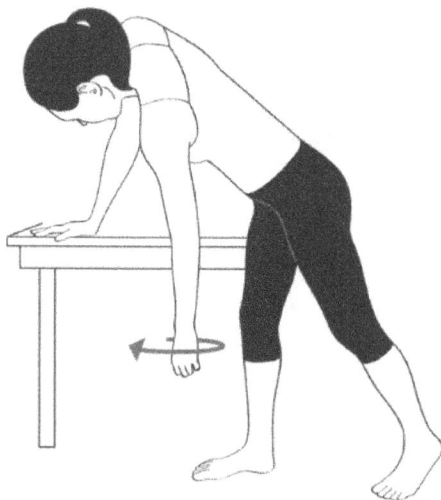

2. Towel Stretch

Hold one end of a small towel behind your back and then grab the opposite end with your other hand.

Hold the towel in a horizontal position.

Next, with your good arm, pull the affected arm upward to stretch it.

You can also do an advanced version of this exercise with the towel draped over your good shoulder.

Hold the bottom of the towel with the affected arm and pull it toward the lower back with the unaffected arm.

Repeat ten to twenty times a day.

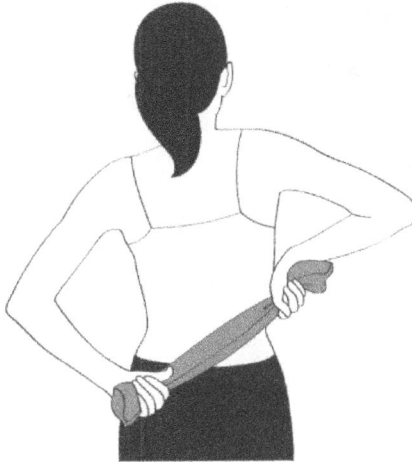

3. Finger Walk

Stand facing a wall, about 6 to 8 inches away.

Reach out and touch the wall at waist level with the fingertips of the affected arm.

With your elbow slightly bent, slowly walk your fingers up the wall, like a stealthy spider, until you've raised your arm as far as you comfortably can.

Slowly lower your arm (assist with your good arm, if you need to) and repeat.

Perform this exercise ten to twenty times a day.

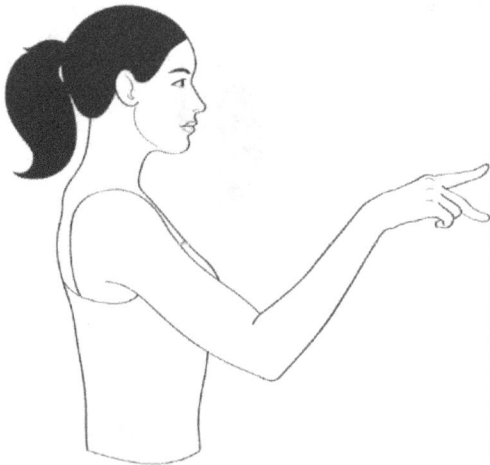

4. Cross-Body Reach

Using your good arm, lift your affected arm at the elbow, and move it up and across your body.

Apply gentle pressure to stretch the shoulder.

Hold the stretch for 15 to 20 seconds. Repeat ten to twenty times per day.

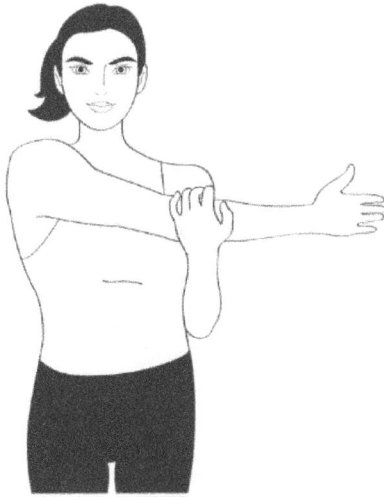

5. Armpit Stretch

Using your good arm, help lift your affected arm onto a shelf about chest level.

Gently bend your knees, opening the armpit. Bend your knees slightly, gently stretching the armpit, and then straighten.

With each knee bend, stretch a little farther, but be careful not to force it.

Repeat ten to twenty times each day.

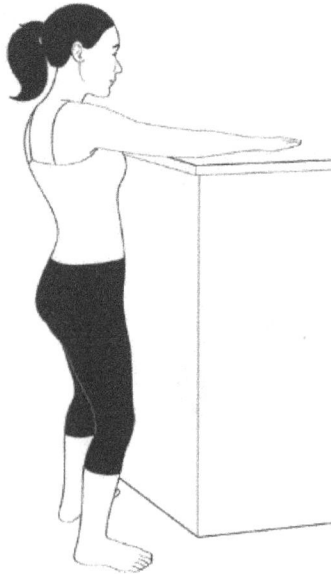

When to Add Rotator Cuff Strengthening Exercises?

As your range of motion improves, add the following two rotator cuff strengthening exercises.

Be sure to warm up your shoulder and do your stretching exercises **before** you perform these strengthening exercises.

6. Outward Rotation

Hold a resistance band loop between your hands with your elbows at a 90-degree angle close to your sides.

Rotate the lower part of the affected arm outward 2 or 3 inches and hold for 5 seconds.

Repeat ten to fifteen times, once a day.

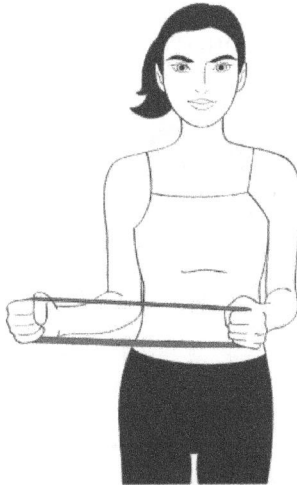

7. Inward Rotation

Stand next to a closed door. Hook one end of a resistance band loop around the doorknob.

Hold the other end with the hand of the affected arm, holding your elbow at a 90-degree angle.

Pull the resistance band toward your body 2 or 3 inches and hold for 5 seconds.

Repeat ten to fifteen times, once a day.

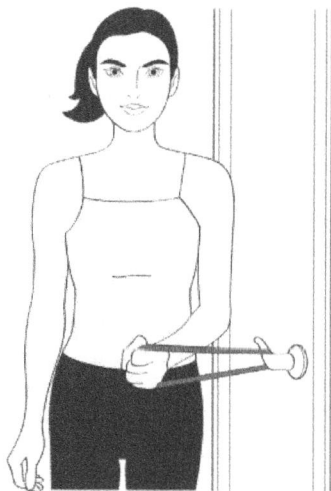

Thoughts

After taking in all this information, it's clear that it takes time to thaw a frozen shoulder. You need patience and a plan. Leaving your shoulder to heal on its own without therapeutic intervention will only result in a painstakingly slow recovery.

Sources

https://www.ncbi.nlm.nih.gov/pmc/articles/PMC4363808/

https://www.mayoclinic.org/diseases-conditions/frozen-shoulder/symptoms-causes/syc-20372684

https://orthoinfo.aaos.org/en/diseases--conditions/frozen-shoulder

https://www.health.harvard.edu/shoulders/stretching-exercises-frozen-shoulder

THE SITTING DISEASE
AND BACK PAIN

Numerous studies have proven that being sedentary can actually have a more dangerous impact on your body than a habit such as smoking would have.

The more hours you sit, the more you increase your chances of developing a serious disease, such as diabetes or cancer.

You're also at greater risk for heart attacks, higher blood pressure, and depression.

It even has its own label—the sitting disease. But to many that's old news, so numerous people are changing to standing desks.

Despite all the new ergonomic furniture that's on the market, there are still those people who need to clock countless hours of seated screen time.

And knowing this information can be frustrating.

Because some people have to sit for multiple hours in order to get their jobs done.

Like G.I. Joe used to say, "Knowing is half the battle." In this case, I mean knowing how to reverse the damaging effects of prolonged sitting (especially with bad posture).

HOW CAN SITTING TOO MUCH CAUSE BACK PAIN?

Sitting for too long causes your low back muscles and hip flexors (the muscles that allow you to lift your knees and bend at your waist) to become short and tight.

Slumped over in a chair all day also makes your abdominal muscles slowly lose tone and your glutes (also known as the buttocks) to become overstretched and weak.

Another phenomenon that happens with prolonged sitting is that it causes an anterior (or front) tilt, which is an adaptive shortening of the hip flexor muscles.

When moving from a prolonged sitting position to an upright one, the shortened hip flexors inevitably pull on the muscle attachments of the lumbar (low back) spine, causing an anterior shift in the hips.

This can put unwanted strain on the low back, exaggerate the lumbar curve, and potentially cause a bulging or herniated disc.

Prolonged lumbar lordosis can also result in back strains or back spasms.

What Is a Back Spasm, and Why Does It Happen?

Back spasms are painful and debilitating, and they can turn a good day into a nightmare.

A back spasm occurs when the low back muscles involuntary tense up or contract in response to protecting themselves from injury.

Back spasms can be caused by arthritis in the back or a ruptured spinal disc. More common reasons for back spasms are from heavy lifting and strenuous physical activities that repeatedly twist and torque the back muscles and ligaments.

Weak abdominal muscles (also known as the core) can make your back more susceptible to injury. Also weak and/or tight back muscles have a higher chance of being injured than stronger and more limber ones.

DOCTOR-RECOMMENDED TREATMENTS

When a back strain or spasm occurs, there are a number of doctor-recommended treatments, such as the following.

Taking muscle relaxants, such as Flexeril. Muscle relaxants should be taken only for a short time to help reduce potential pain flare-ups. It's important to be aware of the common risks and side effects.

Applying hot/cold therapy, such as a reusable gel hot/cold pack or performing an ice massage.

Walking 10 minutes on a treadmill or at a self-selected speed

Using antiinflammatory medication, such as nonsteroidal antiinflammatory drugs (NSAIDs), like ibuprofen and naproxen, which can lead to accidental overdose.

Prolonged drug use can be dangerous to a person's cardiovascular health, carrying severe side effects, such as gastrointestinal and kidney damage.

HOW TO TREAT AND PREVENT FUTURE BACK SPASMS

Once the back spasm has subsided and the pain has fizzled, it's important to do lower back exercises at home to prevent future spasms from creeping back into your life.

So, what are the best lower back pain exercises that will stretch and strengthen your back, so a back spasm won't happen in the first place?

When self-treating low back pain, you'll want to focus on stretching what is tight and strengthening what is weak.

This is based on Sherrington's law of reciprocal innervation, which states that when one muscle is shortened or tightened, its opposite muscle relaxes.

Not everyone has 15 to 30 minutes to do exercises for lower back pain relief, even though it can be tremendously rewarding to find a series of exercises that have been highlighted by back pain doctors as the go-to back pain treatment at home.

That said, here are nine effective lower back exercises you can do at home that will prevent future back spasms from catching you off guard.

NINE EXERCISES TO HELP ERASE LOW BACK PAIN

The following routine should take approximately 10 minutes.

1. Static Hamstring Stretch

Before you begin to rehab your back, spend some time loosening your hamstrings (the tendons at the back of your knee).

Tightness in the hamstrings limits the motion in your pelvis, which can stress the lower back and make it more difficult to stand upright.

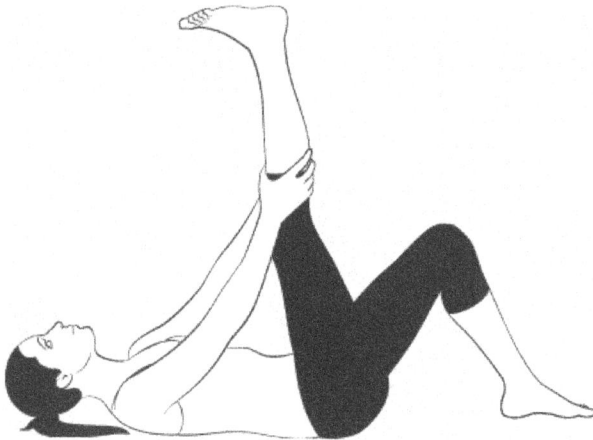

Lie on your back on a firm surface, not a bed.

Grab the back of your leg with both hands.

Pull your leg toward you gently, while keeping both hips on the floor. Hold for 30 seconds.

Repeat two times for each leg.

Contract your abdominals when moving your legs up.

2. Knees to Chest Stretch

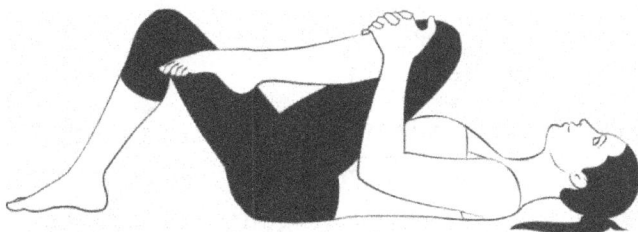

While you're on your back, with your knees bent, grasp your left knee and pull it to your chest.

Hold for 20 seconds.

With your abdominals contracted, try to straighten your right leg.

If you experience any discomfort in your back, leave your right leg bent.

Repeat this move with the other leg.

3. Piriformis Stretch (Lying Down)

The piriformis is a tiny, pear-shaped muscle deep in the glutes that helps laterally rotate the hip.

If it gets too tight, it can impinge the sciatica nerve in the lower back that runs through or under it, causing tremendous pain, tingling, and numbness through the glutes and into the lower leg.

This condition is called piriformis syndrome.

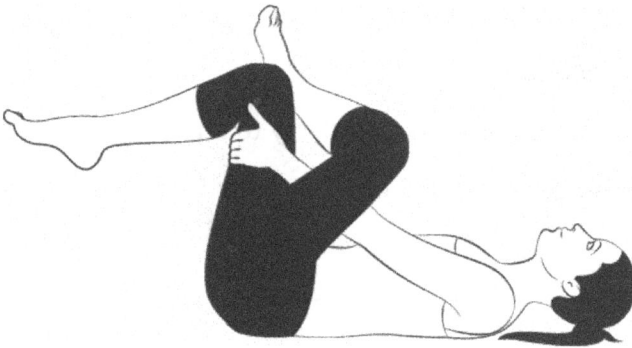

When performing the piriformis stretch, make sure to contract your abdominals before crossing your leg and resting your foot on the other knee.

Hold this stretch for 30 seconds.

Repeat with your other leg.

4. Hip Flexor Stretch

The psoas is the only muscle in the human body connecting the upper body to the lower body. It attaches to the vertebrae of the lower spine, moves through the pelvis, and connects to a tendon at the top of the femur.

A functioning psoas muscle creates a neutral pelvic alignment, stabilizes the hips, supports the lower spine and abdomen, supports the organs in the pelvic and abdominal cavity, and gives you greater mobility and core strength.

Due to the predominant, sedentary culture we live in, most people's psoas muscle is chronically tight, pulling on the muscle attachments of the lower back. This can cause an imbalance in the pelvis that can ultimately lead to severe back pain or even a herniated disc.

By doing this hip flexor stretch, it can help to reverse this phenomenon.

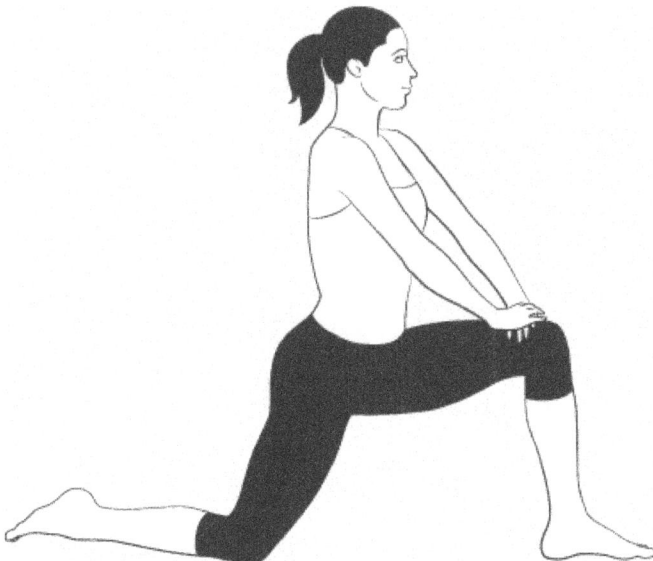

To effectively stretch the hip flexors, first kneel on your right knee, with toes down, and place your left foot flat on the floor in front of you.

Place both hands on your left thigh and press your hips forward until you feel a good stretch in the hip flexors.

Contract your abdominals and slightly tilt your pelvis back while keeping your chin parallel to the floor.

Hold this pose for 20 to 30 seconds.

Then switch sides.

5. Quadriceps Lying Down Stretch (Contract-Relax Version)

Sitting for long periods of time puts the quadriceps muscles (thighs) in a constant contraction, keeping them short and tight.

Stretching the quads will help to prevent this forward flexed posture in the hips and balance the lower back muscles.

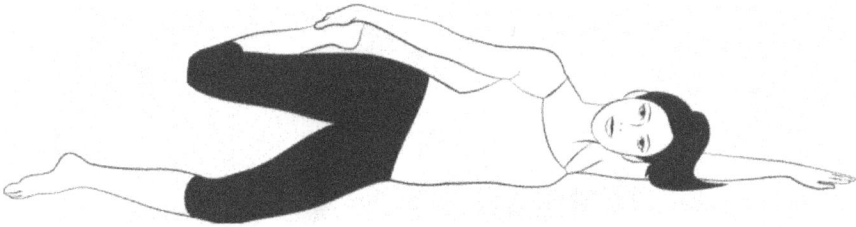

Lie on your side and contract your abdominals, before grasping the top of your foot and moving your ankle toward your glutes.

Hold the stretch for 10 seconds.

For 6 seconds, attempt to straighten your leg, but let your hands "win."

Then relax and stretch your heel toward your glutes for 30 seconds.

6. The Front Plank

Sitting for long periods of time can weaken a person's core muscles. Weak core muscles ultimately diminish a person's natural lumbar curve, creating a scenario for crippling back pain.

This is why doing plank exercises is so vital to your core and back health.

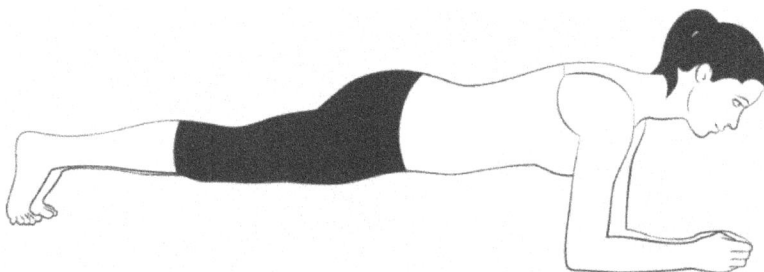

Get into a plank position on the floor with feet hip-width apart and elbows directly under your shoulders.

Brace your core by contracting your abs and attempt to move your belly button toward your spine.

Keep your back straight and legs and glutes engaged the entire time.

Hold this pose for 1 minute.

If 15 to 30 seconds is all you can do, that's fine, just stay at it. The plank exercise works the transverse abdominus. This helps you sit up straight, hold your shoulders back, and prevent forward head posture.

You might feel sore but stay at it and in time you'll be able to work your way up to 1 minute.

7. The Side Plank

When performing the side plank, start by lying on your side with your forearm on the floor under your shoulder to prop you up, and then stack one foot on top of the other.

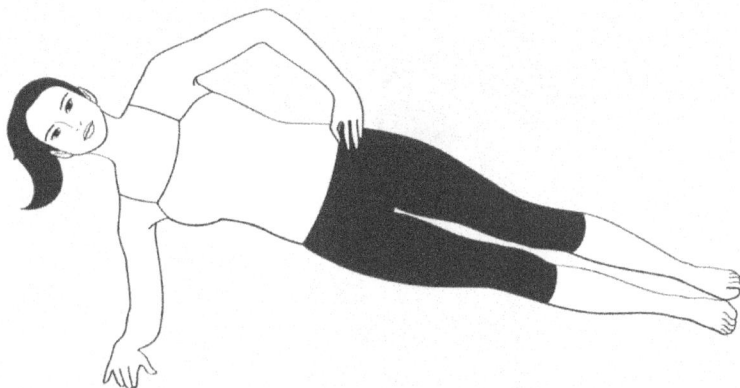

Contract your abdominals and press your forearm into the floor to raise your hips, so that your body is straight from your ankles to your shoulders.

Hold this position for 30 to 60 seconds

Repeat on the other side.

8. Bird Dog

The bird dog (also known as the kneeling superman/superwoman) is a great core and spinal stabilization exercise, as it helps to reinforce proper spinal alignment and strengthen the core.

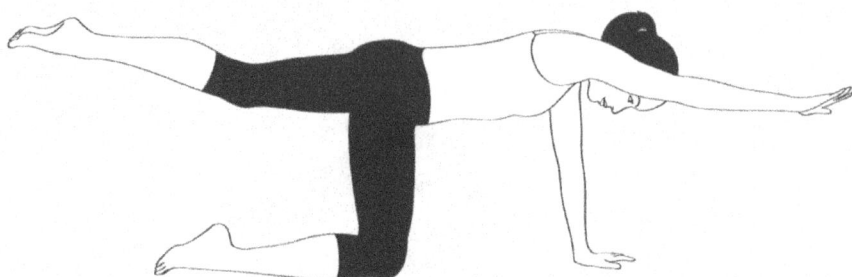

Starting on the all-fours position, tighten your hamstrings, glutes, and lower back. Lift to straighten your leg and opposite arm while maintaining proper alignment.

Perform six, 10-second holds on each side (do all your holds on one side, and then switch sides).

Rest for 20 seconds.

Then perform four, 10-second holds on each side.

9. Glute Bridge

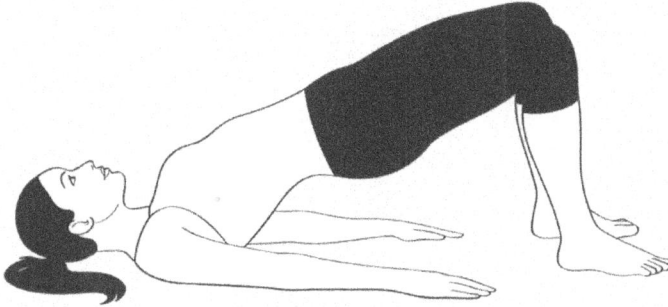

The bridge pose helps to reverse excessive shortening of the hip flexors from prolonged sitting. It helps open and stretch your tight hips, and it also helps strengthen the glutes.

Lie on your back with your hips and knees bent to 90 degrees with your feet flat on the floor and arms by your sides with your palms down.

Take a deep breath in. As you breathe out, lift your hips off the floor until shoulders, hips, and knees are in a straight line.

Hold this pose for 2 seconds and repeat fifteen to twenty times.

DISCOVER ALL THE EXERCISES THAT MELTED AWAY MY BACK PAIN

You should now be experiencing noticeable pain relief and improved flexibility and mobility in your lower back and hips.

These are just some of the exercises I performed every day to heal my back after I injured it one hot summer day installing a 60-pound air conditioner.

If you'd like to discover **all** the exercises that made me feel like my old limber self again, then check out my book, *The Essential Lower Back Pain Exercise Guide.*

I never imagined I'd ever get back pain. But I did, and I learned a wealth of information to overcome it. I've done the hard work of finding all the best exercises and stretches, so you don't need to waste your time looking for what works best.

- You don't need a fancy gym to do these exercises.
- You don't need to see a physical therapist two or three times per week.
- You don't need to buy any costly back pain relief machines.
- You don't need to purchase an ergonomic chair or special shoe inserts.
- You don't need to wear a Velcro back belt. Those don't work!

All you need is a mat or a comfortable surface (not a bed), such as a rug or a carpet, and that's it. In addition, you need the determination and willpower to do the exercises.

I did them every day for twenty-one days, and *boom*—my back pain vanished. I felt stronger than I did before.

My back pain became a distant memory, but I had this vibrant enthusiasm to share these exercise routines with anyone who had back pain, so they could obtain the same relief.

Regular exercise *prevents* back pain. Doctors might recommend exercise for people who have recently hurt their lower backs, suggesting they start with gentle movements and gradually build up the intensity. Once the immediate pain goes away, an exercise plan can help keep it from coming back.

> *"Exercises . . . may be an effective way to speed recovery from chronic or subacute low back pain. . . . Maintaining and building muscle strength is particularly important for persons with skeletal irregularities."*
>
> —National Institute of Neurological Disorders and Stroke

In *The Essential Lower Back Pain Exercise Guide*, you will discover the following essential concepts to prevent or relieve your back pain.

- Nine common back pain myths
- Four most common causes of back pain
- How to stand correctly in six moves
- How to sit correctly in eight moves
- A twenty-one-day, twenty-exercise, 30 minutes-or-less routine

- The 15-minute, doctor-recommended back pain relief routine
- Seven resistance band exercises for low back pain
- Six foam rolling moves to conquer back pain
- Ninety-second, tennis-ball method for low back pain relief
- Six-minute emergency treatment that's safe for herniated and bulging discs
- Seven exercises to prevent future back spasms and herniated discs
- The right way to sleep if you have low back pain
- Four moves to do before you roll out of bed

Thoughts

If you can make time to do a daily, 15 to 30-minute back pain relief exercise routine, you'll soon be on your way to feeling good again. It's essential to feel your best to make the most of every day. Let me show you how!

REFERENCES

Introduction

https://www.thegoodbody.com/back-pain-statistics/

https://www.painscience.com/articles/self-massage.php

Upper Crossed Syndrome and How to Fix It

https://www.ncbi.nlm.nih.gov/pubmed/31040591

https://www.healthline.com/health/upper-crossed-syndrome

Three Postural Stresses That Mess Up Your Shoulders

McKenzie, Robin. *Treat Your Own Shoulder*. 2009.

Upper Crossed Syndrome Exercise Routine

https://www.ncbi.nlm.nih.gov/pmc/articles/PMC5684019/

McKenzie, Robin. *Treat Your Own Neck*. 2011.

McKenzie, Robin. *Treat Your Own Shoulder*. 2009.

https://www.youtube.com/watch?v=prjxXR87Kaw

https://www.youtube.com/watch?v=bMkp_0BtLQg

https://drjohnrusin.com/why-foam-rolling-doesnt-do-what-you-think-it-does/

https://www.msn.com/en-ph/health/exercise/strength/serratus-chair-shrug/ss-BBtOiMP

Bent over L

http://www.coreperformance.com/knowledge/movements/ls-bent-over.html

Bent over Thoracic Rotation

https://www.youtube.com/watch?v=NF9OwEYu1JE

Prone YTW Exercise

https://www.youtube.com/watch?v=3MxHX9j15BU

Correct Rounded Shoulders with These Seven Resistance Band Exercises

https://www.ncbi.nlm.nih.gov/pmc/articles/PMC4932046/

https://www.huffpost.com/entry/frozen-shoulder_b_1733786

http://www.performancehealthacademy.com/thera-band-loop-lat-pull-down.html

https://www.youtube.com/watch?v=4tpl-huz060

https://www.youtube.com/watch?time_continue=24&v=BW0Olzz otBI

Lat Pull Down

http://www.performancehealthacademy.com/thera-band-loop-lat-pull-down.html

Resisted External Rotation

https://www.youtube.com/watch?v=4tpl-huz060

How to Melt Stubborn Knots between the Shoulder Blades

https://www.youtube.com/watch?v=yY-7CXAHxfY

http://backpainok.com/blog/foam-roller-exercises-for-upper-back-and-shoulder-pain/

https://www.doyouyoga.com/6-yoga-poses-to-correct-rounded-shoulders-and-relieve-pain-53703/

Towel Stretch

http://www.functionalsportstherapy.com/resetting-text-neck/

Static Hamstring Stretch

http://www.stretching-exercises-guide.com/hamstring-stretches.html

Knees to Chest Stretch

http://healthyliving.azcentral.com/single-knee-chest-exercise-do-14228.html

Piriformis Stretch (Lying Down)

http://www.spine-health.com/conditions/sciatica/piriformis-muscle-stretch-and-physical-therapy

Hip Flexor Stretch

Ferris, Tim. *The Four-Hour Body: An Uncommon Guide to Rapid Fat-Loss, Incredible Sex, and Becoming Superhuman.* Harmony, 2010.

Quadriceps Lying Down Stretch (Contract-Relax Version)

http://www.knee-pain-explained.com/quadricep-stretches.html

The Front Plank

https://greatist.com/fitness/perfect-plank

The Side Plank

http://www.womenshealthmag.com/fitness/basic-workout-side-plank

http://www.menshealth.com/exercise/side-plank

Bird Dog

http://plankpose.com/bird-dog/

Glute Bridge

https://redefiningstrength.com/best-glute-exercise-glute-bridge/

ABOUT THE AUTHOR

Since becoming a professional massage therapist in 2000, Morgan Sutherland has consistently helped thousands of clients manage their back pain with a combination of deep tissue work, cupping, and stretching. In 2002, he began a career-long tradition of continuing study by being trained in Tuina—the art of Chinese massage—at the world-famous Olympic Training Center in Beijing, China.

As an orthopedic massage therapist, Morgan specializes in treating chronic pain and sports injuries and helping restore proper range of motion. In 2006, Morgan became certified as a medical massage practitioner, giving him the knowledge and ability to work with physicians in a complementary healthcare partnership.

When he's not helping clients manage their back pain, he's writing blog posts about pain relief and self-care, in addition to teaching live and virtual workshops on how to incorporate massage cupping into a bodywork practice. Morgan has received the Angie's List Super Service Award for 2011, 2012, 2013, 2014, and 2015.

Morgan welcomes all comments about your real-life experiences implementing the stretches and exercises contained within this book. Thank you for reading.

Website: www.morganmassage.com
Email: morgan@morganmassage.com

OTHER BOOKS BY MORGAN SUTHERLAND, L.M.T.

The Essential Lower Back Pain Exercise Guide: Treat Low Back Pain at Home in Just Twenty-One Days

Reverse Bad Posture Exercises: Fix Neck, Back, and Shoulder Pain in Just 15 Minutes per Day (Reverse Your Pain Book 1)

Reverse Pain in Hips and Knees: Super-Effective Back, Hip, and Knee Stretches and Strengthening Exercises (Reverse Your Pain Book 2)

Best Treatment for Sciatica Pain: Relieve Sciatica Symptoms, Piriformis Muscle Pain and SI Joint Pain in 20 Minutes or Less per Day

This Is How to Fix Bad Posture: The Best Exercises for Bad Posture That Your Mother Never Taught You

Resistance Band Workouts for Bad Posture and Back Pain: Step-by-Step Illustrated Resistance Band Workouts for Back Pain Sufferers

Twenty-One Yoga Exercises for Lower Back Pain: Stretching Lower Back Pain Away with Yoga

The Essential Massage Cupping Guide : Step-by-Step Cupping Instructions for Treating Chronic Pain & Sports Injuries

DIY Low Back Pain Relief: Nine Ways to Fix Low Back Pain So You Can Feel Like Yourself Again

www.ingramcontent.com/pod-product-compliance
Lightning Source LLC
Chambersburg PA
CBHW060249030426
42335CB00014B/1634